SMASH THAT STUBBORN BELLY FAT

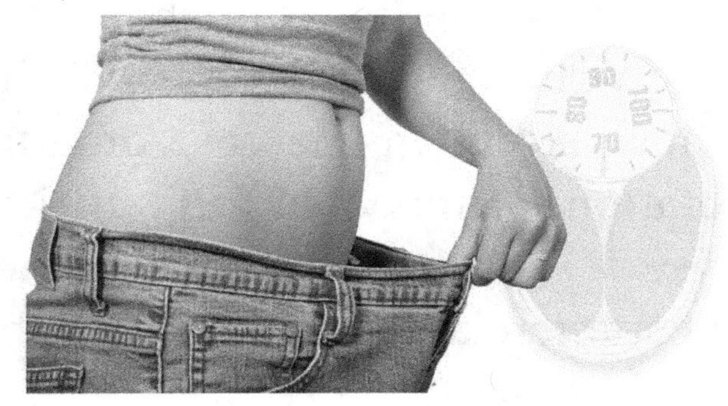

The Ultimate Guide To Melt & Flatten Big Stomach Once & For All

Thelma Pauley

Table of Contents

Introduction

Chapter 1. Understanding Belly Fat:
-Setting Reasonable Expectations

Chapter 2. The Impact of Diet on Belly Fat Loss
-Creating the Perfect Meal Schedule
-How to Balance Macronutrients
-Contemplative Eating
-The Importance of Consistency
-Superfoods that Aid Weight Loss
-Dealing with Cravings and Emotional Eating
-How to Spot Emotional Eating

Chapter 3. Targeted Workouts for a Toned Tummy
-Understanding the Fundamentals
-Core Exercises That Work
-Understanding Cardiovascular Exercise's Role
-Developing a Well-Balanced Fitness Routine

-Ab Workouts for All Levels

-Pilates and Yoga for Core Strength

Chapter 4. Lifestyle Adjustments for Belly Fat

Chapter 5. Supplements to Enhance Your Journey

Chapter 6. Tracking Progress: From Measurements to Photos

Chapter 7. Staying Motivated and Overcoming Plateaus

Chapter 8. Real-Life Success Stories

Conclusion

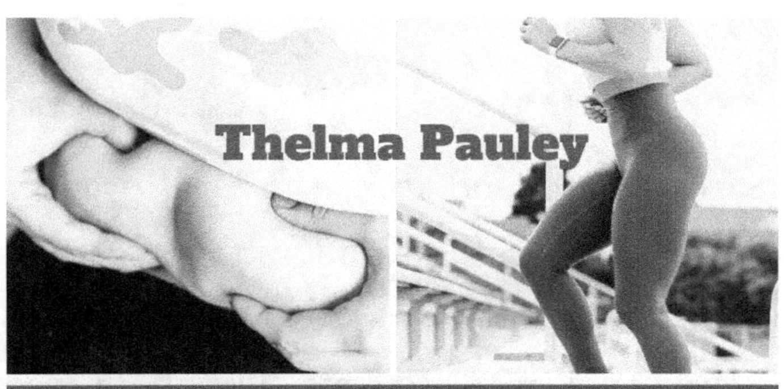

SMASH THAT STUBBORN BELLY FAT

The Ultimate Guide To Melt & Flatten a Big Tummy Once & For All

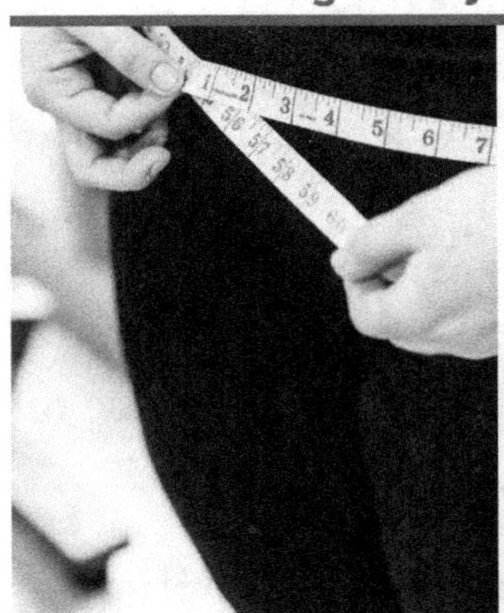

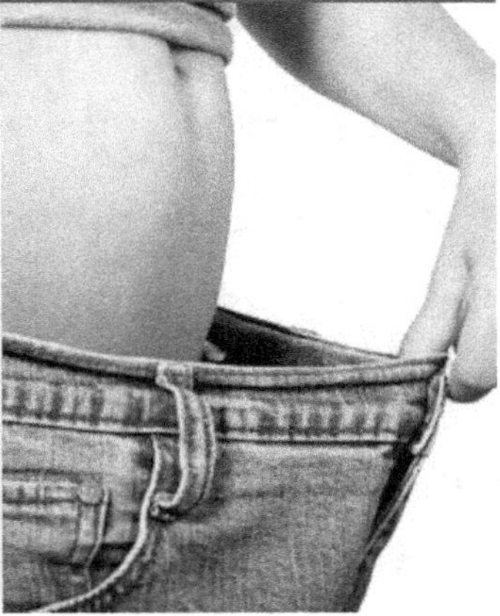

Introduction

Sarah is a friend from the local grocery store. She's just like you and me, leading a busy life with work, family, and the never-ending to-do lists. But there was one thing that was weighing her down, quite literally—her stubborn belly fat.

Sarah had tried it all. She'd experimented with trendy diets, swallowed mysterious pills, and even attempted some of those "get a flat belly in 7 days" challenges she found online. But every time, it felt like her efforts were in vain. The belly fat clung on as if it had a permanent lease on her midsection.

One sunny afternoon, while sipping on her coffee at the local café, Sarah's friend, Lisa, excitedly shared a discovery.

You should take a look at this book I came across, Sarah! It's called 'Smash That Stubborn Belly Fat: The Ultimate Guide to Melt & Flatten Big Stomach Once and for All.'"

Intrigued, Sarah decided to give it a go. She wasn't an expert in fitness or nutrition, and she certainly didn't have hours to spend at the gym. What drew her to the book was the promise of a solution that felt attainable, a way to tackle her belly fat without extreme measures or impossible demands.

As she flipped through the pages, Sarah found a sense of relief. It was as though the author understood her struggles personally. The book didn't promise a magical overnight transformation; it spoke about real challenges and provided real answers. The words on those pages seemed to say, "Hey, we get it. Belly fat is tough. But together, we can conquer it."

Sarah was encouraged to learn about the science behind belly fat, the practical meal plans, and exercises that didn't require a personal trainer. What set this book apart was its accessibility. It was written in plain, straightforward language, as if a friend was guiding her through the journey.

This was the turning point for Sarah. She realized that smashing that stubborn belly fat wasn't a distant dream but a practical goal she could achieve. The book became her trusty companion, offering guidance, motivation, and a sense of belonging to a community of individuals fighting the same battle.

The battle against stubborn belly fat is one that many of us have fought, just like Sarah did. It's a relentless struggle that can feel overwhelming, disheartening, and, at times, even impossible.

But here's the good news: You're not alone, and there is a way forward. "Smash That Stubborn Belly Fat: The Ultimate Guide to Melt & Flatten a Big Stomach Once & For All" is here to empower you with the knowledge and tools you need to win this battle once and for all.

In a world filled with quick fixes and one-size-fits-all solutions, it's easy to feel lost and frustrated in your quest for a flatter, more toned midsection.

I understand the challenges you face, the conflicting advice you encounter, and the ups and downs of trying to shed that belly fat. This book was created with you in mind, offering a comprehensive and realistic approach to achieving your goals.

What should you expect from this treasure book, "Smash That Stubborn Belly Fat"?

1. Science-Backed Strategies:

I dug deep into the science of belly fat to give you an evidence-based plan. You'll obtain a thorough grasp of how belly fat develops all the factors that influence its storage, and the most efficient methods for getting rid of it.

2. Simple Meal Plans:

Quit strict diets and calorie counting. Our book provides easy-to-follow meal ideas that are not only nutritional but also long-lasting. You'll discover how to make eating decisions that will help you lose belly fat.

3. Specific Workouts:

There is no point in spending hours at the gym. We've compiled a list of efficient, focused activities that can help you lose weight. You'll discover workouts to suit your level, whether you're a fitness expert or a novice.

4. Lifestyle Hacks:

Belly fat is caused by more than just what you eat and how you exercise; it is also caused by your general lifestyle. Learn the importance of things such as sleep, stress management, and hydration in your quest for a flatter tummy.

5. Motivation and Overcoming Plateaus:

We'll walk you through the usual problems you'll experience along the way and give you the skills you need to stay motivated and consistent. You'll discover how to overcome obstacles and appreciate

your accomplishments.

6. Actual-Life Success Stories: Throughout this book, you'll read about actual people who fought the same struggle against stubborn belly fat and won. Their experiences and outcomes will motivate you and demonstrate that your objective is feasible.

"Smash That Stubborn Belly Fat" is a support system, a road map, and a source of encouragement. It's a book that recognizes your difficulties while providing a practical, doable road to accomplishment.

As you read on, keep in mind that you're taking an important step toward a better, happier self. Your path to losing stubborn belly fat begins right now, and we'll be there every step of the way.

So, if you've ever felt like Sarah, wishing to say goodbye to that stubborn belly fat, you've come to the correct spot. "Smash That Stubborn Belly Fat" is your traveling companion on your journey.

You'll discover the information, tactics, and motivation you need to make your goal of a flatter stomach a reality in the pages ahead. Allow this book to be your ally as you begin on your journey to permanently eliminate stubborn abdominal fat.

SMASH THAT STUBBORN BELLY FAT

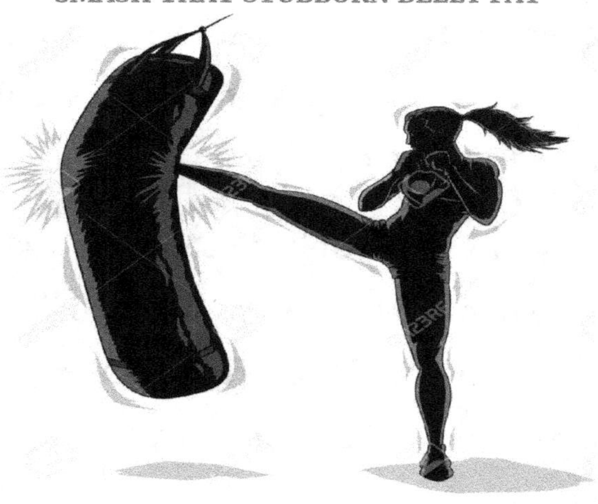

Chapter 1. Understanding Belly Fat: The Key to Smashing Stubborn Belly Fat

Visceral fat, often known as belly fat, is a frequent cause of annoyance for a lot of people. It's that sticky covering of fat that seems to cling to your stomach and accumulate over time.

It can impact not only how you look, but also carries several health dangers. To "Smash That Stubborn Belly Fat," you must first recognize your obstacles.

There are two main types of belly fat: visceral fat and subcutaneous fat. Fat that is directly beneath your skin, or subcutaneous fat, is what you can pinch and feel. Visceral fat is more of a problem, even though it may still be unwanted.

The deep, interior fat that envelops your essential organs, including the pancreas, liver, and intestines, is called visceral fat. Not only does this fat work as insulation, but it is also metabolically active and can produce chemicals and hormones that have a significant effect on your overall health.

Consider that belly fat is an active participant in the complex chemistry of your body, not just a passive lump of padding. To put it simply, this is the lowdown:

1. Where It Hides

Belly fat resides deep within your abdominal cavity, as opposed to subcutaneous fat, which is the fat you can pinch on your thighs or hips. It encircles vital organs such as the pancreas, liver, and intestines. That's right there in the center of things, which is why it's so disturbing.

2. Hormones in Action

Not merely inactive, your belly fat is actively involved. It resembles a tiny factory that produces chemicals and hormones. A few of these may throw off your body's balance. For instance, they may interfere with or lessen the effects of insulin, the hormone that controls blood sugar. They may also trick you into thinking you're more hungry than you are.

3. Inflammation Center

It is well-recognized that belly fat is a hotbed of inflammation. Your body's reaction to dangers, such as infections or wounds, is inflammation. However, it's not a good thing if it persists for a long time. Inflammatory chemicals can be continuously produced by belly fat, and this persistent inflammation has been connected to a variety of health issues, including diabetes and heart disease.

4. The Breakdown of Fat

Another peculiarity of belly fat is that it functions as a small-scale fat burner. Contrary to popular belief, belly fat can break down fat reserves and release fatty acids into circulation. It's as if your body is signaling to you, "I need more energy!" However, if this occurs too frequently, it may interfere with your metabolism.

5. The Fat Around Your Organs

Officially known as visceral fat, this tissue is more than just a passive place to store fat. It is an active, dynamic tissue that is related to every part of your body. It functions similarly to a control center, releasing chemicals and signals that have a variety of effects on your health.

Given everything, what makes it noteworthy, then? That's because belly fat is more than simply a cosmetic concern, according to scientists. It concerns your well-being. It can raise your chance of developing diseases like diabetes and heart disease because of the hormones and inflammation it produces.

Fortunately, the first step to overcoming belly fat is to recognize what kind of fat it is. You can use this knowledge to make wise decisions and "Smash That Stubborn Belly Fat."

We'll cover practical tactics like what to eat, how to exercise, and how to modify your habits in the upcoming chapters. All of it is a necessary step toward being a more positive, happy version of yourself.

Factors Affecting How Much Belly Fat Is Stored

The unwanted friend that sticks to your stomach, belly fat, can be a challenging issue to deal with. To really "Smash That Stubborn Belly Fat," you need to understand the factors that affect how much of it is stored. These components might be compared to a puzzle; once they are put together, you will have a healthier, flatter stomach.

The following are some significant factors impacting the storage of abdominal fat:

1. Genetics

Your body's fat storage location is mostly determined by your genes. You could be more likely to gain excess weight around your middle if your family has a history of doing so. However, lifestyle choices can still have a greater impact than inherited genetic makeup; genetics is not the only factor to take into account.

2. Hormones

Hormones have a significant role in the formation of fat, especially around the abdomen. Two crucial hormones to take into account are cortisol and insulin. Cortisol, also referred to as the stress hormone, can encourage the accumulation of fat around the waist when you are under constant stress. An improper functioning of insulin, the hormone that controls blood sugar, may promote the storage of fat. The key to treating abdominal fat is keeping a balanced hormonal system.

3. Nutrition and Energy Intake

Where your body accumulates fat depends in large part on the foods and calories you eat each day. Consuming too many calories, especially from sugary and high-fat diets, can lead to the buildup of belly fat. Processed foods and sugar-filled drinks are major contributors to weight gain and can generate a lot of belly fat.

4. A Sedentary Lifestyle

The absence of exercise may contribute to the development of belly fat. Regular exercise improves insulin sensitivity, reduces stress, and burns calories. Conversely, visceral fat might develop as a result of a sedentary lifestyle.

5. Getting Older

As we get older, our metabolisms naturally slow down and we tend to lose muscle mass. If our current way of life doesn't change, this could get worse. As we age, maintaining muscle mass with exercise and a healthy diet becomes increasingly important.

6. Stress and Inadequate Sleep

Prolonged stress and insufficient sleep can both affect the buildup of belly fat. Hormone regulation may be impacted by sleep deprivation, leading to heightened hunger and cravings for unhealthy foods. Prolonged stress increases cortisol levels, which can cause the accumulation of belly fat.

First, read "Smash That Stubborn Belly Fat." It explains these components. Each element may interact with the others to create a complex web of effects on your body's accumulation of fat.

However, this intricacy suggests that you have several intervention sites. By adjusting these factors and gradually reducing your belly fat, you can improve your diet, stress reduction, and way of life.

Setting Reasonable Expectations

To truly "Smash That Stubborn Belly Fat," one must have reasonable expectations. Why? You can stay motivated and prevent frustration and disappointment later on by being aware of what is possible and how long it might take.

Here's why success requires having realistic expectations:

1. Being Aware of the Origin of Belly Fat

It's essential that you first understand the

nature of abdominal fat. Visceral fat, another name for this type of fat, is particularly persistent, and significant reductions may take some time. Visceral fat is more resilient and typically one of the last fat reserves to disappear, in contrast to subcutaneous fat, which reacts to dietary and activity changes more quickly.

2. Acknowledging Individual Differences

Because every person's body is unique, the rate at which you lose abdominal fat can vary significantly from person to person. Hormone balance, metabolism, genetics, and general health all come into play. It's important to understand what suits one person and another.

3. Advance at a Reasonable Speed

Recognize that on your path to "Smash That Stubborn Belly Fat," a healthy and sustained weight loss goal typically involves losing 1-2 pounds every week. Quick weight loss is often associated with muscle loss and may lead to health issues. Therefore, strive for patient, consistent improvement rather than quick fixes.

4. Long-Term Dedication Is Essential

Understand that there's more to maintaining and getting a smaller stomach than just a quick fix. It's an investment in your pleasure and well-being for the long run. You are searching for a better way of life that will last over time, not just a temporary solution.

5. Emotional wins

Although the scale's number is one method of measuring development, it's not the only one. Take note of non-scale achievements such as improved sleep, more vitality, greater endurance, and better-fitting clothes. These may provide a more accurate picture of your growth and be more inspiring.

6. Retaining Calm and Resilience

Remember that obstacles and plateaus are normal aspects of the process. It's normal to experience times when the scale stays put or when things are tough for you. During these moments, it is imperative to maintain persistence and patience. It all boils down to consistently making wise choices and adapting your strategy as necessary.

7. Milestone Celebrations

Along the way, give yourself realistic goals or objectives to aim for. Whether it's completing a challenging workout or dropping your first five pounds, acknowledge and celebrate your achievements. Honoring your accomplishments, no matter how modest, can give you a good boost and inspire you to keep going.

In addition to averting needless disappointment, having realistic expectations also encourages a persistent and patient mindset. Recall that the pursuit of "Smashing That Stubborn Belly Fat" is a journey rather than a race. It's about making small, gradual changes over time that pay off in the long run.

If you are willing to make small improvements and have fair expectations, you will be more successful in losing belly fat and reaching your goals.

Chapter 2. The Impact of Diet on Belly Fat Loss

What you eat can make the difference between having that ugly bulge disappear and having a flatter, healthier tummy. Regarding "Smash That Stubborn Belly Fat," diet plays an essential role. As they say, "Abs are made in the kitchen," and there's some truth to that.

Food has a direct impact on your ability to lose belly fat and have a healthy, smaller waist. Let's examine the key elements of how eating might support you in your endeavors.

1. Calorie Management:

Any effective weight loss program must include achieving a calorie deficit. In short, this means consuming fewer calories than your body expels through food. To lose one pound of fat, one must have a calorie deficit of about 3,500. But you must do it healthily and sustainably.

This does not mean that you have to track every calorie exactly. It does, however, entail being aware of your portion sizes and listening to your body's signals of hunger and fullness. You may be able to naturally cut calories while still getting the essential elements you need by selecting meals that are higher in nutrients and lower in calories and by reducing portion sizes.

2. Effectively balanced meals:

Having well-balanced meals is essential to following a healthy diet plan. This means combining dishes from different dietary groups. Every meal should ideally consist of:

- **Protein:** While you're losing weight, lean protein sources like beans, fish, chicken, lean meats, and tofu will help you feel satisfied.

- **Carbohydrates:** Select complex sources of carbohydrates such as fruits, vegetables, and whole grains. They help control blood sugar levels and provide sustained energy.

- **Healthy Fats:** Add foods like avocados, almonds, seeds, and olive oil to your meals as sources of healthy fats. These fats support overall health and satiety.

3. High-quality carbohydrates

When it comes to carbohydrates, the quality is crucial. Choose complex carbohydrates over refined and high-sugar options. Complex carbs include legumes and a variety of vibrant vegetables, as well as whole grains like quinoa, brown rice, and oats. These foods provide you with the essential nutrients, dietary fiber, and steady energy release, so you can feel full without experiencing energy shortages.

4. High-Fibre Foods

When it comes to combating belly fat, fiber is your ally. Meals high in fiber, such as those made with whole grains, fruits, vegetables, and legumes, help to regulate digestion in addition to satisfying appetite. Soluble fiber in particular has been shown to lower visceral fat.

5. Fibre-Lean

Protein is an important factor to consider while trying to lose weight. It helps you burn more calories by maintaining your muscle mass and increasing your metabolic rate. Include lean protein sources in your meals to increase the effectiveness of your diet in reducing the fat around your abdomen.

6. Staying Hydrated

Although it's commonly overlooked, maintaining your fluid intake is crucial to your diet. Our bodies might occasionally mistake thirst for hunger, leading to overindulgence in calories. Throughout the day, staying hydrated will help you control your hunger and prevent overindulging in food.

7. Time of Meal

Although the idea of eating several small meals throughout the day is widely accepted, the most crucial factor to take into account is overall calorie intake. The total number of calories consumed is what counts, regardless of whether you eat three larger meals or several smaller ones.

8. Steer clear of liquid calories

Drinks could be a covert way to consume extra calories. Fruit juices, sugar–filled beverages, and excessive drinking might soon add up. Drink water, herbal tea, or other nutrient-rich, low–calorie beverages to stay hydrated.

9. Mindful Consumption

Eating mindfully is being extremely conscious of what and how much you eat. It means savoring every bite, eating without interruptions from media (such as TV or phones), and paying attention to your body's signals of hunger and fullness. This can help you avoid overindulging and make healthier food choices.

Embracing these dietary recommendations into your daily routine is a key first step in "Smashing That Stubborn Belly Fat." It's crucial to understand, though, that spot reduction—the removal of fat from a specific area—rarely works. Instead, focus on overall fat loss by eating a balanced diet and exercising frequently. Belly fat will gradually disappear as your body sheds excess fat in various areas.

Creating the Perfect Meal Schedule

Many people who want to improve their appearance and health often find themselves wanting to fight against stubborn abdominal fat. Exercise is crucial, but when it comes to getting a flatter and healthier waistline, the proverb "you are what you eat" is very true. A well-crafted meal plan is a crucial part of your strategy for "Smash That Stubborn Belly Fat."

Let's look at how to create a meal plan that fits your goals, provides the calories you need, and promotes fat reduction.

Determining Specific Goals

Setting defined goals is the first step in designing your perfect diet plan. What do you want to achieve in your quest to eliminate abdominal fat? Understanding your goals, whether it's a certain amount of weight loss, a specific waist circumference, or just a healthy midsection, will help you plan your meals.

Caloric Requirements

The foundation of every meal plan is an awareness of your daily calorie requirements. To lose weight effectively, you must create a calorie deficit, which means consuming fewer calories than your body burns. This usually includes reducing your daily calorie intake by 500 calories, resulting in a consistent weight loss rate of 1-2 pounds each week.

Healthy Meals and Snacks

Divide your daily calorie consumption into balanced meals and snacks. Three large meals (breakfast, lunch, and dinner) with two to three smaller snacks in between are a common habit. This helps to avoid bingeing and overeating while also keeping blood sugar levels constant.

How to Balance Macronutrients

Each meal should have a macronutrient balance of protein, carbohydrates, and healthy fats. Protein is necessary for muscle maintenance, carbohydrates for energy, and healthy fats for satiety and overall health.

Protein Prioritization

Protein is vital for achieving your belly fat loss goals. It gives you a feeling of fullness, assists in the retention of lean muscle mass, and can enhance your metabolic rate. Incorporate lean protein sources such as poultry, fish, lean beef, tofu, lentils, and low-fat dairy into each meal.

Choosing High-Quality Carbohydrates

When it comes to carbohydrates, quality matters. Choose complex carbohydrates such as whole grains, fruits, and vegetables over processed and sugary carbohydrates. Complex carbs provide long-lasting energy and assist in blood sugar management.

Vegetable-Rich Meals

When it comes to decreasing belly fat, vegetables are your greatest friend. They are low in calories yet abundant in fiber, vitamins, and minerals. At lunch and dinner, strive to fill half of your plate with vegetables. They thicken your meals and enhance fullness without adding many calories.

Fitness Fats

As sources of healthy fats Include avocados, almonds, seeds, and olive oil in your diet. These fats enhance the flavor of your food and make you feel full.

Contemplative Eating

Pay attention to your body's hunger and fullness cues to practice mindful eating. Eat away from the TV or computer, which can lead to mindless overeating.

Hydration

Staying hydrated is sometimes overlooked, yet it is vital to any dietary regimen. Sometimes our bodies misinterpret thirst for hunger, resulting in excessive calorie consumption. Drinking adequate water throughout the day will help you regulate your appetite and avoid overeating.

Control of Portions

Portion management is essential for preventing overeating. Using smaller dishes may help you reduce portion sizes and avoid overeating.

Adaptability and customization

While the concepts shown above provide a solid basis, keep in mind that your perfect meal plan should be tailored to your specific preferences, dietary restrictions, and lifestyle. Allow for little wiggle space in your diet plan to account for occasional indulgences and alterations.

The Importance of Consistency

Consistently following your well-planned diet plan is crucial to success. The path to gradual and persistent belly fat loss is to constantly establish a calorie deficit while making wise food choices.

We'll go over more meal planning, recipe ideas, and specific dietary alternatives to help you "Smash That Stubborn Belly Fat." With a well-planned meal plan and a clear grasp of beneficial nutritional options, you'll be well-prepared to make smart and successful decisions in your quest for a flatter and healthier stomach.

Superfoods that Aid Weight Loss

In your quest to "Smash That Stubborn Belly Fat," your food may be your most powerful ally. While there is no magical meal that will melt belly fat on its own, incorporating a variety of nutrient-rich superfoods into your diet can help you achieve your belly fat reduction goals.

These superfoods are abundant in vitamins, minerals, fiber, and other nutrients that can aid in weight loss. Let's have a look at some of the superfoods you should include in your diet.

1. Berries:

Antioxidants and fiber are abundant in blueberries, strawberries, and raspberries. Antioxidants combat inflammation, which adds to belly fat, and fiber aids digestion and keeps you satisfied. Berries are a delicious addition to meals, snacks, and smoothies.

2. Fatty Fish:

Omega-3 fatty acids are abundant in fatty fish such as salmon, mackerel, and sardines. These healthy fats can reduce inflammation and accelerate fat loss, particularly in the abdominal area. At least twice a week, include fatty fish in your diet

3. Avocado:

Avocado is a superfood that is abundant in healthy monounsaturated fats that help you feel full and content. They also include a lot of fiber, vitamins, and minerals. Avocado slices go well with sandwiches, salads, and guacamole dip.

4. Quinoa:

Quinoa is a complete grain with a high protein, fiber, and vitamin and mineral content. Its high protein content may help with hunger control, and it's a healthier choice than processed carbs. Quinoa may be used to make salads, side dishes, and even breakfast bowls.

5. Greek Yogurt:

High in protein and probiotics, Greek yogurt aids digestion. It is a substantial and nutritious snack or breakfast alternative due to its high protein content.

6. Leafy Greens:

Low-calorie leafy greens including spinach, kale, and Swiss chard are high in fiber, vitamins, and minerals. They are excellent at promoting fullness and supplying essential nutrients.

7. Nuts and Seeds:

Almonds, walnuts, chia seeds, and flaxseeds are abundant in fiber, protein, and healthy fats. They are a tasty snack that may alleviate hunger while also supplying essential nutrients.

8. Lentils with beans:

Fiber and protein are abundant in beans and legumes such as black beans, lentils, and chickpeas. They help with hunger control and blood sugar regulation. These versatile ingredients may be used in soups, salads, and as a meat substitute in several dishes.

9. Whole Grains:

Whole grains, such as brown rice, oats, and whole wheat bread, contain complex carbohydrates, fiber, and vital nutrients. They give sustained energy and help regulate blood sugar levels, reducing energy crashes and cravings.

10 Green Tea:

Green tea contains catechins, which have been linked to increased fat burning, particularly in the stomach area. Drink a cup of green tea as part of your daily regimen.

11. Eggs:

Eggs are a great source of protein and essential nutrients. Including eggs in your breakfast or meals may help you feel full while reducing weight and maintaining muscle mass.

12. Turmeric:

Curcumin, an active component in turmeric, has anti-inflammatory and antioxidant properties. It may help reduce belly obesity and inflammation. Make a turmeric drink or use it in your cooking.

13. Apples:

Apples are abundant in fiber and water, making them filling. They are a fast and healthy snack that may assist you in controlling your appetite.

14. Lean meats:

Chicken and turkey are high in protein and low in fat. Protein is required for muscle preservation and has the potential to increase metabolic rate.

15. Oatmeal:

Oatmeal is a whole grain that is high in fiber and provides long-lasting energy.

It's an excellent breakfast option for getting your day started correctly.

Remember that, while these superfoods may aid in the loss of belly fat, a well-rounded, balanced diet is also required. Include a variety of these superfoods in your meals and snacks to receive the maximum benefits. When paired with a well-planned diet and regular exercise, these superfoods can help you achieve a flatter and healthier tummy.

Portion Control: Your Eating Plan to Lose Belly Fat

Portion control is an important aspect of healthy eating that may help you manage your calorie intake and achieve your belly fat reduction goals. This post will provide you with amazing insights into portion control and practical methods to help you consume the right amount to help you lose weight.

Understanding Portion Control

Portion control is the practice of consuming a certain amount of food that matches your nutritional needs and weight loss goals. It requires keeping track of how much you consume, whether you dine at home, out, or grab a quick snack. Portion control is used to avoid overeating, control calorie intake, and achieve or maintain a healthy weight.

The Importance of Portion Control

1. Calorie Management:

Portion control helps with calorie management. Consuming more calories than your body requires can lead to weight gain, while maintaining a calorie deficit can lead to weight loss, including the reduction of belly fat.

2. Avoiding Overeating:

In our age of massive portions, it's easy to consume more than your body requires. Overeating can result in discomfort, weight gain, and difficulty with your weight loss goals.

3. Balanced Nutrition:

Portion control encourages a nutritious diet. When you eat in reasonable amounts, you have room for a variety of meals from various food groups, ensuring that your body obtains the nutrients it requires.

Potential Portion Control Methods

1. Use Smaller Dishes:

Using smaller dishes can make portions appear larger, allowing you to feel satisfied with less food.

2. Measuring Instruments:

Invest in measuring cups and a food scale to accurately measure quantities, especially if you're cooking or preparing meals at home.

3. Divide Restaurant Meals:

When dining out, split the entrée or quickly package up part of your meal to avoid overeating.

4. Engage in Mindful Eating: Recognize your body's hunger and fullness signs. Eating slowly and enjoying each meal may help you prevent overeating.

5. Learn visual cues:

Learn to recognize visual cues regarding portion amounts. A serving of lean protein is about the size of a deck of cards, whereas a cup of cooked pasta is around the size of a tennis ball.

6. Single Servings:

Choose single-serving packages or split out food into tiny containers to minimize mindless eating.

7. Begin with smaller portions: Begin with smaller portions and allow yourself to return for more if you're still hungry. This would help to avoid overeating from large initial meals.

8. Avoid Consuming straight from Containers:
Consuming straight from a bag or container may result in overconsumption. Pour a small amount and then trash the container.

9. Mindful Meal Preparation:
Plan your meals and snacks so that you have nutritional options on hand. This assists in avoiding impulsive, large servings.

10. Drink lots of water:

Endeavor to drink a lot of water throughout the day to stay hydrated. Your body might occasionally misinterpret thirst for hunger, resulting in unnecessary calorie consumption.

Dealing with Cravings and Emotional Eating

Controlling cravings and emotional eating are essential for successfully treating persistent abdominal fat. These obstacles frequently lead to the consumption of unhealthy meals, which impedes your weight loss goals. In this article, we'll look at practical techniques to cope with cravings and emotional eating so that you may regain control of your eating habits and get a flatter, healthier stomach.

How to Recognize Cravings

Cravings are strong desires for certain foods, which are typically high in sugar, salt, or unhealthy fats. They can be triggered by a variety of factors, including stress, hormonal changes, or simply seeing or smelling enticing foods. Cravings are natural, but regulating them is essential for losing weight.

How to Spot Emotional Eating

Emotional eating is when instead of facing our emotional pains (stress, anger, or loneliness) head-on, we use food to deal with them. Emotional eating can result in overeating and weight gain.

Emotional Cravings and Eating

1. Be Mindful:

Recognize when you have an emotional hunger or yearning. Consider what motivates your urge for a snack before reaching for one.

2. Distracting Yourself:

Do something distracting for a set length of time, such as 10-15 minutes, while you're hungry. This might frequently help to lessen the craving.

3. Hydration:

Drink a glass of water before succumbing to hunger; because most times we confuse thirst with hunger or vice versa.

4. Healthy Substitutes:

Keep healthful choices on hand for quick treatments. If you crave sweets regularly, have fresh fruit or dark chocolate with a high cocoa content available.

5. Portion Control:

If you want to satisfy your appetite, practice portion control. Instead of overindulging, try a little portion of your favorite meal.

6. Psychological Coping Strategies:

Consider alternatives to eating to cope with emotions. Physical exercise, deep breathing, script, or conversing with a friend might all be examples.

7. Meditative Eating:

To practice mindful eating, take your time with each meal and remove distractions. This may help you appreciate your food more and identify fullness cues.

8. Daily Meals and Snacks:

Eating at regular times will help you prevent feeling hungry, which can contribute to cravings and overeating.

9. Deal with Emotional difficulties: If you're feeling upset or struggling with your emotions, it's a good idea to talk to a doctor or counselor for help.

10. Journaling:

Keeping a food journal to track your cravings and emotional eating may help you detect what prompts and triggers such eating styles.

11. Social Support:

Discuss your goals with friends or family members who can keep you responsible and provide support.

12. Good Stress Management: Incorporate stress-reduction activities into your daily routine, such as meditation, yoga, or hobbies.

Food Links for Health

You must first create a balanced and healthy connection with food to get a flatter stomach and maintain a healthy weight. We know that overcoming cravings and emotional eating can be tough, but the strategies discussed above can help you make better and more meaningful meal choices. Applying these tactics consistently while keeping a regular work pattern will enable you to effectively manage cravings and emotional eating. This development is critical for "Smashing That" stubborn abdominal fat

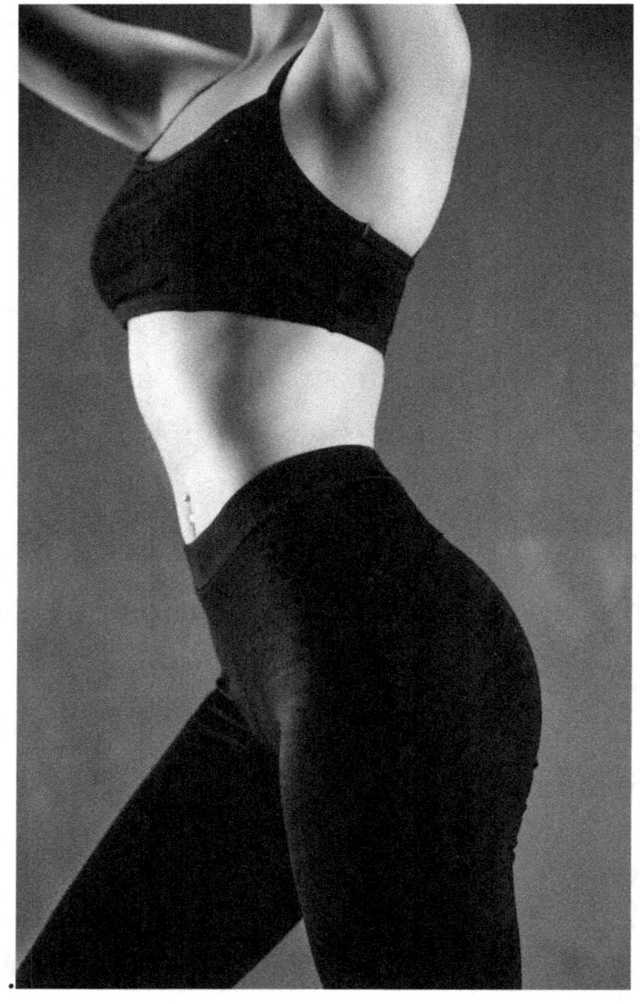

Chapter 3. Targeted Workouts for a Toned Tummy

Exercise is essential in your quest to "Smash That Stubborn Belly Fat," as it tones and strengthens the muscles in your abdominal area. While spot reduction (fat loss in a specific location) is not a practical technique, focused workouts can assist in enhancing muscle tone and definition in your abdomen.

This chapter will walk you through effective stomach toning and strengthening workouts and routines.

Understanding the Fundamentals

Before going into specific routines, it's critical to understand the core muscles that comprise your midsection. Several muscle groups make up the core, including:

1. Rectus Abdominals

These are the muscles that are generally referred to as "abs" and are in charge of flexing your spine.

2. Obliques

The obliques, which run down the sides of your abdomen, aid in twisting and bending actions.

3. Transverse Abdominis

This is the deepest layer of your core muscles, and it functions as a natural weight belt, stabilizing your spine and pelvis.

4. Erector Spinae

These muscles go down your spine and help with core strength and posture.

Core Exercises That Work

1. Crunches:

-Lie on your back with your legs bent and your hands behind your head.

- Raise your head and shoulders off the ground while contracting your abs.

 - Go back to where you began and do it again.

2. Planks:

- Begin in a push-up stance, forearms on the ground.

- Keep your body in a straight line from your head to your toes by using your tummy muscles.

- Hold for as long as you can, trying to become longer with each session.

3. Leg Raises:

Lie on your back and straighten your legs.

- Stretch out your legs and lift them toward the sky.

- Return them to the starting position without letting them contact the ground, then repeat.

4. Russian Twists:

Lie on your back with your knees bent and your feet flat.

- Slightly lean back, maintain your back straight and lift your feet off the ground.

- Twist your torso to the right, then to the left, touching the ground with your hand.

5. Bicycle Crunches

Lie on your back, elevate your head and shoulders, and stretch your right leg while bringing your right elbow toward your left knee.

- Move your legs like you're pedaling a bike, switching sides each time.

6. Bird Dog

Begin in a tabletop position on your hands and knees.

- Bring your right arm forward and your left leg back in a straight line.

- Hold for a few seconds before switching to the other arm and leg.

An Example of a Tummy Toning Routine

- Stay in the plank position without letting your tummy touch the ground for 30 seconds.

- Crunches: three sets of fifteen repetitions.

- Leg Raises three sets of twelve repetitions.

- Russian Twists: three sets of twenty twists (10 on each side).

- Bicycle Crunches: three sets of twenty twists (10 on each side).

- Bird Dog: three sets of ten repetitions (5 on each side).

Remember:

- Consistency is essential. Perform focused core workouts at least twice a week.
- For total fat reduction, combine core exercises with full-body workouts.
- Maintain a nutritious diet to help you achieve your fitness objectives.
- If you're new to exercise or have any medical issues, speak with a fitness professional.

When paired with a healthy diet and an overall fitness regimen, targeted core workouts can help you tone your belly and reach the results you want. In the following chapter, we'll look at the role of cardiovascular activity in losing belly fat.

The secret to effective belly fat reduction exercise is a multifaceted program that involves both strength training and aerobic activity. We'll look at why combining these workouts is important and how to plan your fitness regimen for the best outcomes.

Understanding Cardiovascular Exercise's Role

Cardiovascular exercise, sometimes known as "cardio," is any physical activity that boosts your heart rate and breathing rate. Jogging, swimming, cycling, and brisk walking are examples of such activities. Cardiovascular activity is necessary for belly fat loss for numerous reasons:

1. Calorie Burn: Cardio workouts burn calories, assisting you in establishing a calorie deficit, which is required for fat reduction, particularly belly fat.

2. Fat Loss Throughout the Body: Cardio exercise involves your whole body, boosting general fat reduction. When you expend calories, your body uses stored fat, particularly belly fat, to generate energy.

3. Lowers Visceral Fat: Cardiovascular activity has been demonstrated to lower visceral fat, which is the deep abdominal fat that surrounds your organs and contributes to a wider waistline.

Successful Cardiovascular Exercises

1. Running/Jogging:

Running at a moderate to high effort burns a lot of calories.

2. Cycling:

Biking is a low-impact workout that can be modified to accommodate people of various fitness levels.

3. Swimming:

Swimming is a total-body workout that works your core and burns calories.

4. Aerobics and Dance:

Classes that are fun and active might help you enjoy your aerobic workouts.

5. High-Intensity Interval Training:

HIIT is a type of workout that comprises short bursts of intense exercise followed by brief rest intervals and is extremely effective at burning calories.

Strengthening Exercises

While aerobic activity burns calories and aids in fat reduction, strength training is also essential. Building muscle raises your resting metabolic rate, which means you burn more calories even when you're not moving. Strength training exercises, such as weight lifting or bodyweight workouts, can help shape and define your body while losing fat.

Developing a Well-Balanced Fitness Routine

To effectively decrease belly fat, a well-balanced fitness plan that includes both aerobic activity and strength training is required. Here's how to plan your workouts:

1. Cardiovascular Activity:

Aim for at least 150 minutes of moderate-intensity exercise every week or 75 minutes of high-intensity cardio spaced out across multiple days.

2. Strength Training:

Include strength training exercises targeting key muscle groups 2-3 times per week. For balanced results, focus on your core while simultaneously working on your legs, arms, and back.

3. Recovery and Rest:

Give your body time to recuperate between sessions. Recovery is the process by which your muscles recover and develop stronger.

Example Weekly Fitness Schedule

- Monday:
30 minutes of moderate-intensity cardio (brisk walking).

- Tuesday:

Strength training with an emphasis on the core (e.g., planks, leg lifts).

- Wednesday:

20 minutes of moderate-intensity aerobic cycling.

- Thursday:

Total-body strength exercise (squats, push-ups, etc.).

- Friday:

15 minutes of high-intensity cardio (HIIT).

- Saturday:

Rest or gentle stretching.

- Sunday:

30 minutes of moderate-intensity aerobic swimming.

Remember:

- It is critical to maintain consistency. Maintain your exercise routine for long-term results.

- A well-balanced diet works in conjunction with your exercise efforts to reduce belly fat.

- If required, get expert counsel from a fitness professional.

Both cardiovascular and weight training are excellent methods for reducing abdominal fat. A well-rounded physical plan combined with a healthy diet can assist you in reaching your objectives.

Cardiovascular Exercise Routines

1. Consistent Walking Routine:

- Stretch for 5 minutes as a warm-up.

- Brisk Walk: 30-45 minutes at a pace that raises your heart rate while enabling you to talk.

- 5 minutes of slow-paced walking to cool down.

- Stretching: After your workout, stretch for 10 minutes to enhance flexibility.

2. High-Intensity Interval Training Routine

- Warm-up: 5-10 minutes of easy cardio (for example, running in place).

- HIIT Session: 20-30 minutes of high-intensity activity (for example, sprinting) followed by 30 seconds of rest or low-intensity exercise (for example, walking).

- Cool down with 5-10 minutes of light exercises.

- Stretching: After your workout, stretch for 10 minutes.

3. Cycling Routine:

- **Warm-up:** 10 minutes of gentle cycling.

- 45-60 minutes of moderate to vigorous riding.

- Cool down with 10 minutes of easy cycling.

- Stretching: After your workout, stretch for 10 minutes.

Remember:

- Consult a fitness specialist before beginning any new training routine, especially if you have any underlying health issues.

- To maintain consistency, select workouts that you enjoy.

- Consistency is the key to effective belly fat reduction. Strive for a minimum of

150 minutes of moderate-intensity cardiovascular exercise per week.

Cardio activities will help you get a slim waist. Combine these exercises with a well-balanced diet and targeted core routines for overall belly fat removal. We'll look at how sleep and stress management may help you attain a healthier, flatter belly in the following chapter.

Ab Workouts for All Levels

There are ab workouts that you may integrate into your program regardless of your fitness level. Begin with exercises that are appropriate for your present level and improve as you gain confidence and strength.

Beginner Ab Workouts

1. Crunches:

Lie down on your back with your legs bent and your hands behind your head. Lift your head and shoulders off the ground, then descend back down while activating your abdomen. Repeat for a total of three sets of 15 repetitions.

Leg Raises:

Lie on your back and straighten your legs. Straighten your legs and lift them toward the ceiling. Lower them back down without allowing them to make contact with the earth. A rep for three sets of 12 repeats.

3. Boards:

Begin in a push-up posture, forearms on the ground. Keep your body in a straight line from head to heels by engaging your core muscles.

Intermediate Ab Workouts

1. Bicycle Crunches:

Lie on your back, elevate your head and shoulders, and stretch your right leg while bringing your right elbow toward your left knee. In a pedaling action, alternate sides. Repeat for three sets of 20 reps (10 per side).

2. Russian Twists:

Sit on the ground with your knees bent and your feet flat. Lift your feet off the ground and lean back slightly, keeping your back straight. Twist your torso to the right, then to the left, touching the ground with your hand. Repeat for three sets of 20 twists (10 on each side).

3. Bird Dog:

Begin in a tabletop posture on your hands and knees. Maintain a straight line by extending your right arm forward and your left leg back. Hold for a few seconds before switching to the other arm and leg. Repeat for three sets of ten repetitions (5 on each side).

Advanced Ab Workouts:

1. Leg Raises While Hanging:

Lift your legs straight up toward the ceiling while hanging from a pull-up bar. Return them to the ground without swinging. A rep for three sets of 12 repeats.

Dragon Flags:

Lie on a bench or a sturdy surface with your head over the edge. Lift your legs and lower your body while maintaining your back straight. Return your body to the beginning position. A rep for three sets of ten repetitions.

Plank Variations:

Plank variations such as side planks,

forearm planks, and raised planks will test

your core.

Tips for Insane Ab Workouts

- To avoid injuries, warm up before your ab workouts.

- Maintain perfect form during each exercise to adequately activate your core.

- Maintain consistent breathing throughout your repetitions, exhaling as you exert effort.

- Increase the intensity or duration of your workouts progressively as your core strength develops.

Include these ab exercises in your workout program and modify the effort level to your current level of fitness. Developing a strong core is an important part of your route to a leaner, healthier midsection. The importance of diet in your belly fat reduction objectives will be discussed in the next chapter.

Pilates and Yoga for Core Strength

In your quest to "Smash That Stubborn Belly Fat," mind-body techniques such as yoga and Pilates can be game changers. These practices provide distinct approaches to core strength, flexibility, and general well-being. In this chapter, we'll look at the benefits of yoga and Pilates for core strength and how they may help you on your way to a leaner, healthier midsection.

Yoga: A Comprehensive Approach to Core Strength

Yoga is a centuries-old discipline that incorporates physical postures, breathing methods, meditation, and awareness. It focuses on strengthening the bond between the body and mind by encouraging balance, flexibility, and core strength.

Yoga for Core Strength Advantages

1. Better Posture:

Yoga promotes body awareness and stimulates the core muscles, resulting in better posture and less stress on the lower back.

2. Core Functional Strength:

To increase functional strength, several yoga postures target the core muscles, such as the rectus abdominis, obliques, and transverse abdominis.

3. Flexibility:

Yoga improves flexibility, which can aid in core engagement during other workouts and lower the chance of injury.

4. Reduced Stress:

Yoga's mindfulness and deep breathing practices will help you minimize stress and emotional eating, which can aid in your belly fat loss quest.

5. Balanced Muscle growth:

Yoga encourages balanced muscle growth, which is critical for lowering the risk of muscular imbalances and injury.

Key Core Strength Yoga Poses

1. Plank:

Planking engages your whole core, including the front, sides, and back. Hold this stance for at least 30 seconds.

2. Navasana (Boat Pose):

The rectus abdominis is strengthened in this sitting stance. Lift your legs and upper body off the ground while remaining balance on your sit bones.

3. Setu Bandhasana (Bridge Pose):

This backbend strengthens the core while engaging the glutes and lower back.

4. Adho Mukha Svanasana (Downward Dog):

As you support your weight on your arms and shoulders, you activate the entire body, including the core.

Key Pilates Exercises for Core Strengths

1. Hundred:

This exercise involves controlled breathing and pumping your arms while engaging your core muscles.

2. Leg Circles:

Leg circles work the lower abdominals and hip flexors, improving core stability.

3. The Saw:

The saw involves twisting and stretching, targeting the obliques and core muscles.

4. Swan Dive:

The swan dive strengthens the erector spine and back muscles, complementing core strength.

Incorporating Yoga and Pilates into Your Routine

To enjoy the benefits of yoga and Pilates for core strength, consider the following tips:

1. Choose Your Style:

There are various styles of yoga and Pilates, so explore different classes or videos to find the one that resonates with you.

2. Frequency:

Aim to practice yoga or Pilates 2-3 times a week, complementing your existing fitness routine.

3. Mindfulness:

Both practices emphasize mindfulness and proper breathing. Focus on your breath and form during each session.

4. Consistency:

Like any exercise, consistency is key. Make yoga and Pilates a regular part of your routine.

5. Professional Guidance:

If you're new to these practices, consider taking classes or working with a certified instructor to ensure proper form and technique.

6. Progression:

As you become more experienced, challenge yourself with more advanced poses and exercises to continually build core strength.

Yoga and Pilates offer holistic approaches to core strength, flexibility, and mental well-being. Incorporating these practices into your fitness routine can enhance your journey to a leaner and healthier midsection. In the next chapter, we'll delve into the importance of nutrition and how it supports your belly fat reduction goals.

Chapter 4. Lifestyle Adjustments for Belly Fat

In this chapter, we'll look at the key lifestyle changes that may make a big impact in your quest for a leaner, healthier stomach. It's not only about exercise and food when it comes to losing belly fat; it's also about building a sustainable and supportive atmosphere for your objectives.

Making wise lifestyle choices will increase your chances of success and guarantee that your progress is sustainable. We'll walk you through the holistic adjustments that will help you accomplish your ultimate goal, from sleep and stress management to mindful eating and hydration.

So, let's delve into these critical changes that will allow you to regain control of your body and produce long-term benefits.

1. Stress and Sleep Management

Adequate sleep and stress management are sometimes ignored yet critical components of belly fat reduction.

- **Sleep:** Try to get 7-9 hours of undisturbed sleep each night. Sleep deprivation can affect hormones that control hunger, leading to overeating and weight gain, particularly in the abdomen.

- **Stress Reduction:** Chronic stress might result in an increase in abdominal fat. To keep stress at bay, use stress-reduction practices like meditation, deep breathing, or yoga.

2. Hydration

Hydration is important for general health

and can help with hunger management. Drinking plenty of water can help you distinguish between thirst and hunger, keeping you from overeating.

3. Dietary Balance

Maintain a nutritious diet that includes fruits, vegetables, lean meats, whole grains, and healthy fats. Avoid sugary beverages, processed meals, and trans fats, which can all lead to belly obesity.

4. Portion Management

Take note of portion sizes. Excessive consumption of even nutritious meals might result in weight gain. To help manage servings, use smaller plates and utensils.

5. Routine Meals

Meal timing must be consistent. Have regular, balanced meals during the day to keep your energy stable and avoid overeating later on.

6. Avoid Consuming Liquid Calories

Calories from sugary beverages such as soda, fruit juices, and energy drinks add up rapidly. Opt for water, herbal tea, or other low-calorie drinks instead.

7. Mindfulness in Eating

Savor your meal and pay attention to hunger and fullness signs to practice mindful eating. While eating, avoid distractions such as devices.

8. Maintain Physical Activity

Include physical activity in your daily routine.Non-exercise activities such as walking, gardening, or using the stairs can all help you burn calories.

9. Social Assistance

Involve friends or family members on your adventure. Sharing your objectives and progress with a support network can help to motivate and hold you accountable.

10. Patience and Consistency

It takes time to lose belly fat. Maintain your workout and diet regimen and be patient with the process.

11. Monitoring Progress

Maintain a log of your exercises, food, and improvements. Tracking can assist you in identifying patterns and making required changes.

12. Setting Goals

Set attainable goals and appreciate your accomplishments. Smaller goals might help enhance motivation.

13. Professional Counseling

Consider seeking tailored advice and assistance from a healthcare practitioner or a certified dietician.

14. Self-Care

Make self-care a priority to minimize stress and increase overall well-being. This might include hobbies, relaxing techniques, or enjoyable activities.

15. Avoid Snacking Late at Night

Late-night eating might contribute to weight gain. Attempt to complete your meals at least a couple hours before going to bed.

16. Reduce Alcohol Consumption

Alcohol contains a lot of empty calories. Reduce your alcohol consumption to help your weight reduction objectives.

17. Give up smoking

Quitting smoking can enhance your overall health and lower your risk of visceral fat formation.

18. Maintain Your Knowledge

Continue your education in nutrition,

fitness, and wellbeing. Staying educated allows you to make better decisions.

Making these lifestyle changes will help you achieve your goals of losing belly fat and keeping a healthy stomach. By implementing these modifications into your daily routine, you will be well on your way to reaching your fitness and health objectives.

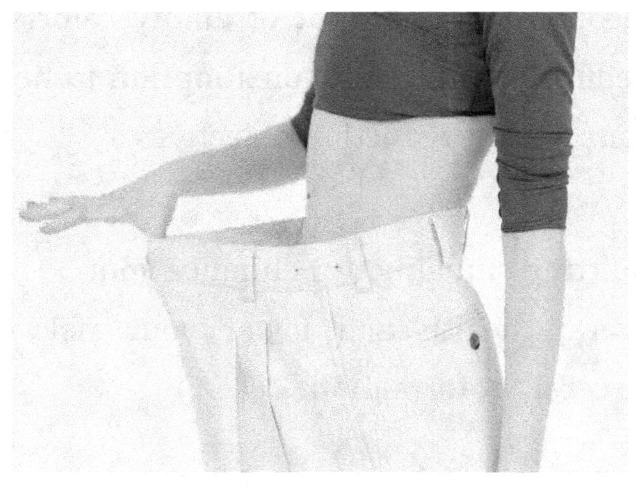

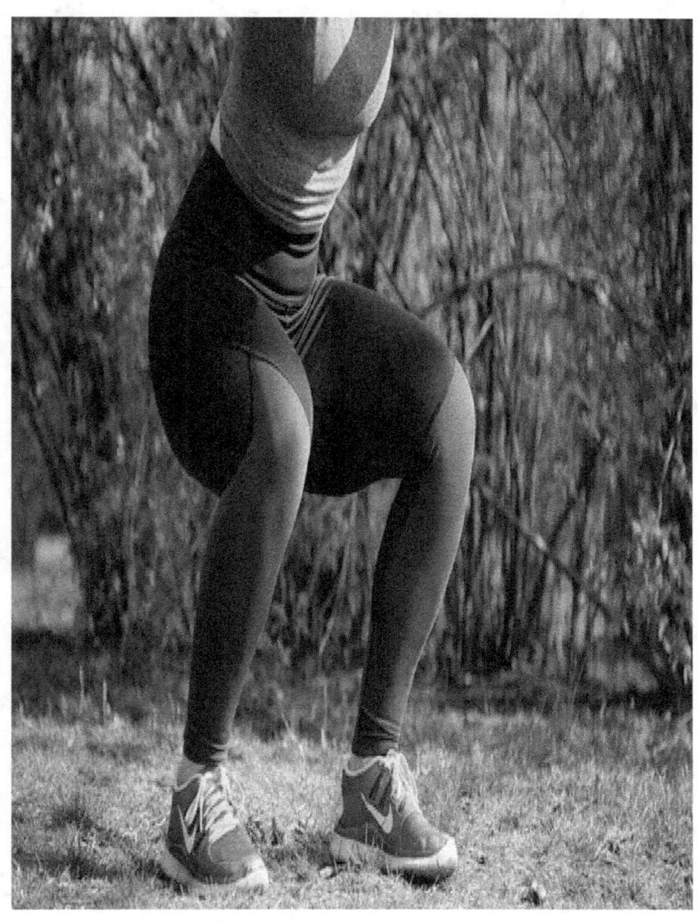

Chapter 5. Supplements to Enhance Your Journey

Supplements might be a valuable complement to your overall plan. While supplements are not a substitute for a well-balanced diet and regular exercise, they can deliver certain nutrients and chemicals that help you achieve your fat reduction and health objectives.

In this chapter, we'll look at various vitamins that might help you have a leaner, healthier stomach.

Please keep in mind:

Before incorporating any supplements into your regimen, speak with a healthcare practitioner or qualified dietitian to confirm they are appropriate for your specific requirements and health state.

1. Multivitamins:

A high-quality multivitamin can help you address dietary gaps in your diet by providing key vitamins and minerals for general health and metabolic function.

2. Omega-3 Fatty Acids:

Omega-3 supplements, which are often derived from fish oil or algae, can aid in the reduction of inflammation and the maintenance of cardiovascular health, both of which are vital in any fat-loss journey.

3. Vitamin D:

Vitamin D is important for fat metabolism and general health. If your levels are low, a supplement may be useful.

4. Fiber Supplements:

Fiber supplements can aid with digestive

health and appetite management by producing a sensation of fullness.

5. Probiotics:

Probiotic pills help improve gut health, which can have an influence on weight loss and metabolism.

6. Green Tea Extract:

Green tea extract includes chemicals such as EGCG, which may aid in fat oxidation and metabolism.

7. Caffeine:

Caffeine pills can boost alertness and energy, potentially improving athletic performance.

8. CLA (Conjugated Linoleic Acid):

CLA supplements are thought to help in fat reduction by altering the body's metabolism.

9. Glucomannan:

Glucomannan is a kind of fiber that can aid with appetite management by providing a sense of fullness.

10. Prebiotics:

Prebiotic pills can encourage the growth of healthy gut bacteria, which can improve general health and perhaps aid in weight loss.

11 Branched-Chain Amino Acids (BCAAs):

BCAA supplements can help with muscle maintenance during calorie restriction or strenuous exercise, which is essential for fat reduction.

12. Iron:

Iron supplements may be required, particularly for women suffering from iron deficiency anemia. Iron is involved in energy metabolism.

13. Protein Powder:

Protein supplements can help you get enough protein, which is necessary for muscle maintenance and hunger management.

14. L-Carnitine:

L-carnitine supplements are considered to help fatty acid transport into the mitochondria of the cell, where they may be utilized for energy.

15. Chromium:

Chromium supplements are occasionally used to help with blood sugar regulation, which can affect food and desires.

Remember:

Supplements are supposed to supplement, not replace, a balanced diet and lifestyle. Prioritize a healthy diet, frequent exercise, and lifestyle aspects such as sleep and stress management. Supplements should be taken cautiously and in collaboration with a healthcare practitioner to ensure they are appropriate for your unique objectives and needs.

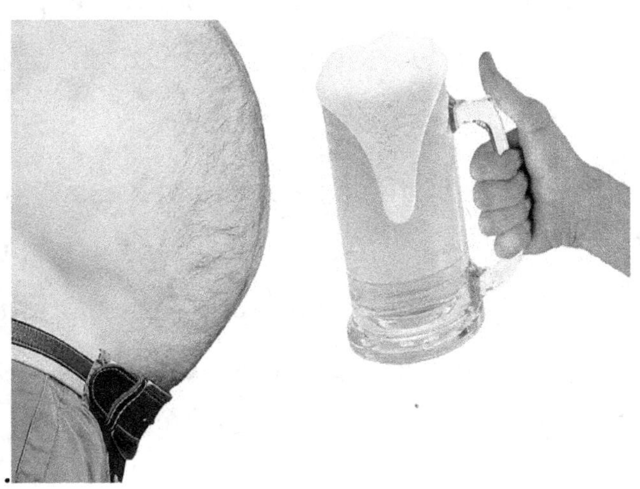

Chapter 6. Tracking Progress: From Measurements to Photos

Monitoring your progress is crucial for your success in losing belly fat. Tracking your accomplishments not only gives encouragement, but also useful insights into what is working and where changes may be required.

This chapter discusses the necessity of documenting your progress, from collecting measurements to taking images, and shows you how to do so efficiently.

Why Tracking Progress Is Important

1. Motivation:

Seeing your progress can help you stay motivated and on track toward your goals.

2. Accountability:

Tracking makes you responsible to your goals and helps you stick to your fitness and diet plan.

3. Identifying Trends:

By recording your journey, you will be able to spot patterns and trends in your outcomes and make better decisions.

4. Modification and Adaptation:

Tracking enables you to determine what needs to change in your approach if you reach a plateau or face problems.

Progress Tracking Methods That Work

1. Measurements:

Take regular measurements of your waist, hips, and other pertinent areas.

- Take measurements on a regular basis, such as weekly or monthly, to observe changes over time.

2. Weight:

While not the only sign of improvement, the scale can give insights into overall patterns.

- To minimize variances, weigh oneself at the same time of day and under consistent settings.

3. Shots:

Take full-body shots from various perspectives that are inconsistent with lighting.

- Side by side photo comparisons might indicate noticeable changes in your body.

4. Body Fat Percentage:

If feasible, determine body fat percentage using technologies such as skinfold calipers or bioelectrical impedance.

- Body composition changes are frequently more significant than weight changes.

5. Fitness Examinations:

To perform fitness examinations, such as timed runs, strength tests, or flexibility measurements, to analyze physical performance gains.

6. Food and Exercise Logs:

- Maintain an accurate record of your regular food consumption and exercise regimens. This can assist you in identifying links between your behaviors and your outcomes.

Tips for Efficient Progress Monitoring

1. Be Consistent:

For measurements, pictures, and evaluations, use the same methodology, instruments, and circumstances.

2. Use Several Metrics:

To assess success, avoid depending entirely on one metric (e.g., weight). Combining measurements, photographs, and fitness tests results in a more complete picture.

3. Set Specific objectives:

Establish clear and realistic objectives for what you want to achieve so that you can measure your progress more easily.

4. Appreciate Milestones:

To stay motivated, acknowledge and appreciate your accomplishments along the path.

5. In progress Check-Ins:

Track progress at regular intervals, but avoid daily assessments because natural swings can be deceiving.

6. Patience:

Recognize that growth is not always linear

and that plateaus or setbacks are common.

The Influence of Visualization:

It may be really encouraging to see your progress through measurements and images. It helps you to see how far you've come and motivates you to keep going. Remember that change takes time, and keeping track of your progress will help you remain on track toward your ultimate goal of a leaner, healthier midsection.

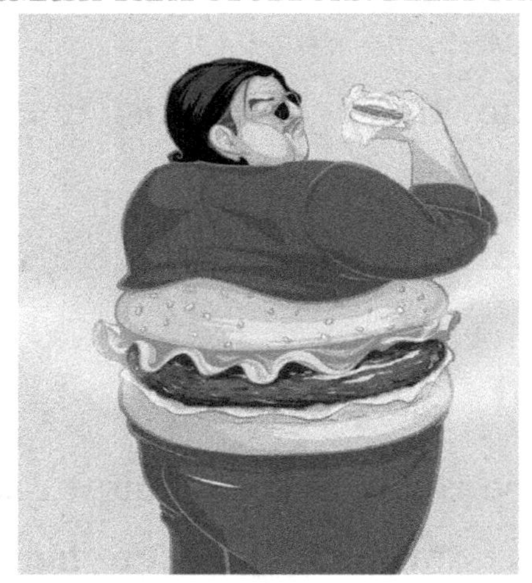

Chapter 7. Staying Motivated and Overcoming Plateaus

Keeping motivated and coping with plateaus are unavoidable aspects of the process. This chapter will provide you the skills and methods you need to keep your excitement going and overcome those difficult moments of stagnation.

The Value of Motivation

Your growth is propelled forward by motivation. It's what pulls you out of bed in the morning for your workout and keeps you eating well. Maintaining motivation, on the other hand, can be difficult, especially when faced with challenges such as plateaus.

Motivational Strategies

1. Set defined, quantifiable objectives: Having defined, quantifiable objectives provides you with a feeling of purpose and direction.

2. Visualize Success:

Picture yourself attaining your objectives. Visualization may be a very effective motivator.

3. Appreciate Small Wins: Acknowledge and appreciate even the most minor accomplishments along the road.

4. Remain Accountable:

Share your objectives with a friend or exercise partner who can help you stay on track.

5. Change Your Routine:

Variety may rekindle your passion. Experiment with different exercises, diets,

and fitness challenges.

6. Track Your Progress:

Measure your progress on a regular basis and utilize visual aids such as images to show how far you've come.

7. Seek Help:

Join a fitness community or locate a mentor who can offer advice and motivation.

8. Keep Informed:

To keep involved, educate yourself about diet, exercise, and general health on a regular basis.

9. Remember Your "Why":

Go back over your reasons for going on this trip and utilize them as inspiration.

Overcoming Obstacles

Plateaus are prevalent in fitness and can be discouraging. They are, however, not a dead end; rather, they are a task to conquer. Here's how it's done:

1. Modify Your Routine:

Change your workout and eating routine. Change your workout program, raise the intensity, or try different meals to shake your body out of its rut.

2. Set New Goals:

Refocus your efforts by establishing new goals that will push you in new ways.

3.Mindful Eating:

Pay strict attention to your diet. Mindful eating can assist you in identifying trends and making better choices.

4. Rest and Recovery:

Your body requires a break from time to time. Check to see whether you're receiving adequate rest and sleep.

5. Remain Consistent:

Maintain your regimen even when improvement slows. Plateaus are not always permanent.

6. Seek Professional Advice:

If you're having trouble, consult with a fitness professional or a dietician.

The Mindset Effect

Motivation and overcoming plateaus are both dependent on your mentality. Maintain an optimistic attitude, recognize that setbacks are inevitable, and keep your ultimate aim in mind.

Remember that your trip is about more than simply getting to your destination; it's about the change and growth you go through along the way. In the following chapter, we'll look at how to keep your momentum going by practicing portion control and mindful eating, two crucial components of your approach to "Smash That Stubborn Belly Fat."

Common Challenges in Achieving Weight Loss and Ways to Conquer Them

In your journey to "Smash That Stubborn Belly Fat," you will face a variety of weight reduction difficulties that will put your dedication and commitment to the test. Understanding these problems and developing solutions to overcome them is critical for long-term success. Let's examines several frequent roadblocks and offer strategies to overcome them.

1. Plateaus:

Challenge:

Plateaus are times of halted development in which your weight or body fat appears to be frozen.

Solution:

Adjust your routine, increase intensity, tweak your nutrition, and be patient to break through plateaus.

2. Emotional Eating:

Challenge:

Stress-related or emotional eating might disrupt your dietary strategy.

Solution:

Recognize emotional triggers, practice mindfulness, and develop healthy stress coping strategies.

3. Cravings

Challenge:

Cravings for unhealthy meals might be difficult to overcome.

Solution:

To avoid cravings, choose healthier choices, exercise portion control, and remain hydrated.

4. Lack of Motivation:

Challenge:

Motivation might decrease, making sticking to your fitness and eating plan tough.

Solution:

To enhance motivation, revisit your goals, imagine success, celebrate minor victories, and seek assistance.

5. Peer Pressure:

Challenge:

Social gatherings and peer pressure can contribute to unhealthy eating habits.

Solution:

Plan ahead of time, express your intentions to friends and family, and surround yourself with supportive social groups.

6. Time Restrictions:

Challenge:

Exercise and healthy food preparation can be difficult to fit into busy schedules.

Solution:

Prioritize time management, schedule efficient exercises, and plan nutritious meals ahead of time.

7. Doubt about Oneself:

Challenge:

Self-doubt may stymie development and cause you to abandon your ambitions.

Solution:

Maintain a good attitude, focus on your accomplishments, and remember why you began your trip.

8. Injuries and Medical Problems:

Challenge:

Injuries or medical conditions might disturb your workout schedule.

Solution:

Consult a healthcare expert, make

necessary adjustments to your workout routine, and prioritize rehabilitation.

9. Irrational Expectations:

Challenge:

Unrealistic aspirations can lead to despair and disappointment.

Solution:

Set precise, attainable goals and applaud achievement along the way.

10. Deficit of Information:

Challenge:

Success might be hampered by a lack of information about nutrition and exercise.

Solution:

Continue to learn, seek expert advice, and be educated about health and wellness.

11. Boredom

Challenge:

Boredom can be caused by monotonous routines, lowering motivation.

Solution:

Change up your workout routine, try different healthy dishes, and find joy in your journey.

12. Overtraining:

Challenge:

Excessive exertion without adequate rest might result in burnout and injury.

Solution:

Rest and recuperation should be prioritized, as well as active recovery days.

13. Quick Solutions:

Challenge:

Falling for fad diet or supplement claims of quick weight loss.

Solution:

Recognize that long-term improvements require time, and concentrate on sustainable, healthy techniques.

Overcoming these frequent weight reduction obstacles needs tenacity, patience, and a willingness to adapt. By identifying and tackling these roadblocks, you'll be more able to remain on track and eventually achieve your goal of a leaner, healthier midsection.

In the following chapter, we'll look at portion management and mindful eating, two critical components of your approach to "Smash That Stubborn Belly Fat."

Chapter 8. Real-Life Success Stories

In the quest to "Smash That Stubborn Belly Fat," understanding the science and strategies is crucial, but drawing inspiration from real-life success stories is equally vital. This chapter is dedicated to sharing the remarkable journeys of everyday people who conquered their belly fat, showcasing the power of dedication, healthy habits, and the drive to change.

Success Story 1: Sarah's Remarkable Journey

Sarah, a devoted mother with a full-time job, faced the common challenge of reclaiming her pre-pregnancy body amidst a hectic lifestyle. What sets

Sarah's journey apart is her unwavering commitment.

Despite juggling work and family responsibilities, she embraced a balanced diet and incorporated regular exercise into her routine. Over the course of a year, Sarah's dedication resulted in a remarkable 40-pound weight loss. Her journey exemplifies the strength and resilience that can emerge from a determined mindset.

Success Story 2: John's Transformation from Desk to Fitness

John's story resonates with many working professionals who find themselves grappling with the consequences of a sedentary job.

Frustrated with his physical condition, John took decisive action.

He introduced a consistent exercise routine and adopted a balanced diet, showcasing the transformative power of lifestyle changes. Over two years, John shed an astonishing 60 pounds, demonstrating the significant impact of discipline and regularity in achieving enduring results.

Success Story 3: Emily's Postpartum Progress

For new mothers like Emily, navigating postpartum weight loss can be especially challenging. What makes Emily's journey noteworthy is her pragmatic approach. Focusing on short, effective home workouts and embracing a balanced postpartum nutrition plan, Emily lost 30 pounds in a year. Her story emphasizes the importance of setting attainable goals and recognizing the unique demands of each life phase.

Success Story 4: Mark's Midlife Transformation

Mark's decision to prioritize health in his mid-40s challenges the notion that age is a barrier to change. By incorporating strength training and modifying his diet, Mark achieved a remarkable 50-pound weight loss over two years. Mark's journey serves as a beacon for those who may hesitate due to age-related concerns, proving that positive transformations are achievable at any stage of life.

Success Story 5: Lisa's Journey to a Balanced Lifestyle

Lisa, a college student, provides a perspective on the significance of balance in health and fitness. By adopting a holistic approach to nutrition and exercise, Lisa not only shed 25 pounds but also fostered a healthier relationship with her body and food. Her story underscores the importance of mental well-being and self-compassion in the pursuit of overall fitness.

Drawing Inspiration from Real-Life Triumphs

These inspiring narratives collectively emphasize that anyone, regardless of their circumstances, can embark on a transformative journey. The common threads among these individuals are dedication, consistency, and a willingness to adapt.

As you pursue your own goal to "Smash That Stubborn Belly Fat," draw motivation from these real-life triumphs. Remember that your journey is unique, and with commitment, you too can script a success story that inspires others.

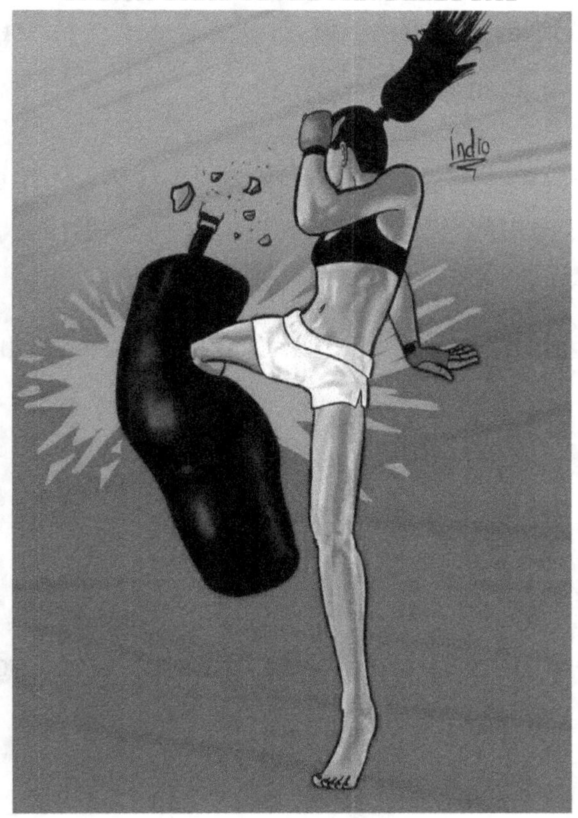

Conclusion

You've finished this thorough book after exploring an extensive collection of ideas, effective techniques, and real-life success stories, all created to aid your journey toward a flatter tummy.

Beyond the physical, this pursuit implies a significant adjustment in lifestyle, habits, and overall well-being. As we conclude, let us summarize the major points and define essential techniques for your continued success.

Progress Reflection

This guide has been an in-depth study of the essential elements of your transformational journey:

1. Understanding Belly Fat

Discovered the science underlying belly fat, its causes, and the challenges of losing it.

2. Factors Influencing Belly Fat Storage

Examined the effects of heredity, hormones, and lifestyle decisions on belly fat formation.

3. Establishing Realistic Expectations

Highlighted the essential role of achievable goals as the basis for success.

4. Successful Nutrition Strategies

Understood the value of balanced meals, portion control, and mindful eating.

5. Diet's Role in Belly Fat Loss:

Looked into the relationship between nutrition, fat reduction, and the effect of macronutrients.

6. Creating Your Ideal Meal Plan

Discovered how to design a tailored meal plan based on goals and interests.

7. Superfoods to Help You Lose Weight

Introduced several superfoods to help with metabolism and weight reduction.

8. Portion Control

Stressed the significance of portion control as a technique for calorie management.

9. Tackling Cravings and Emotional Eating

We spoke about how to cope with cravings and emotional eating.

10.Targeted Workouts for a Toned Tummy

Studied workouts that tone and strengthen the core.

11. Effective Exercise for Belly Fat Loss

Recognized the need for efficient, focused workouts.

12. Cardio Workouts for a Slimmer Midsection

You learned about the function of aerobic exercises in calorie burning.

13. Specific Ab Exercises for All Levels

Investigated a variety of ab workouts appropriate for varied fitness levels.

14. Full-Body Workouts to Increase Calorie Burn

The need for full-body training for general fat reduction was emphasized.

15. Yoga and Pilates for Core Strength

Introduced low-impact methods to strengthen and stretch the core.

16. Lifestyle adjustments for Belly Fat Success

Looked into lifestyle adjustments that support fitness objectives.

17. The Role of Sleep and Stress Reduction

The importance of sleep and stress reduction in weight loss was emphasized.

18. The Effect of Staying Hydrated on Fat Loss

The impact of water on metabolism and health was discussed.

19. Supplements to Help You Along the Way

Considered potential supplements to supplement fitness and diet routines.

20. Tracking Progress: From Measurements to Photos

Recognized the need for progress tracking for motivation.

21. Strategies for Overcoming Weight Loss Obstacles

Provided insights and methods for dealing with challenges.

22. Developing Healthy Habits for Long-Term Success

The significance of developing and keeping healthy behaviors was discussed.

23. Celebrating Success and Maintaining Outcomes

Investigated the relevance of recognizing accomplishments and maintaining outcomes.

24. Inspiring Accounts of Those Who Overcame Recalcitrant Belly Fat

Take inspiration from real-life success stories.

Your Next Steps

Remember that the route to a flatter stomach is more than just outward looks. It is about improving one's health, self-esteem, and general quality of life. To secure long-term success:

1. Create precise, measurable, and achievable goals.

2. Maintain a consistent approach to exercise, nutrition, and lifestyle behaviors.

3. Continue to document progress using measurements, pictures, and performance measures.

4. Be willing to change routines as your body and goals change.

5. Continue to study about diet, exercise, and general health.

6. To keep motivated and accountable, share your goals with a supportive community.

7. Recognize and reward yourself as you reach milestones.

8. Be kind to yourself, accept that setbacks may occur, and remain devoted to your goals.

9. Concentrate on long-term outcomes through lasting lifestyle adjustments.

10. Reflect on your development and draw inspiration from real-life success tales.

In essence, the trip to a flatter stomach is one-of-a-kind, packed with hurdles and triumphs. Accept the process, enjoy your accomplishments, and continue on your path to a healthier, fitter, and more confident self.

Your success is a continuous process of growth and progress, not a destination. Imagine yourself in a better state, and may the road ahead be full of pleasure, joy, and the blessings of a life well-lived.